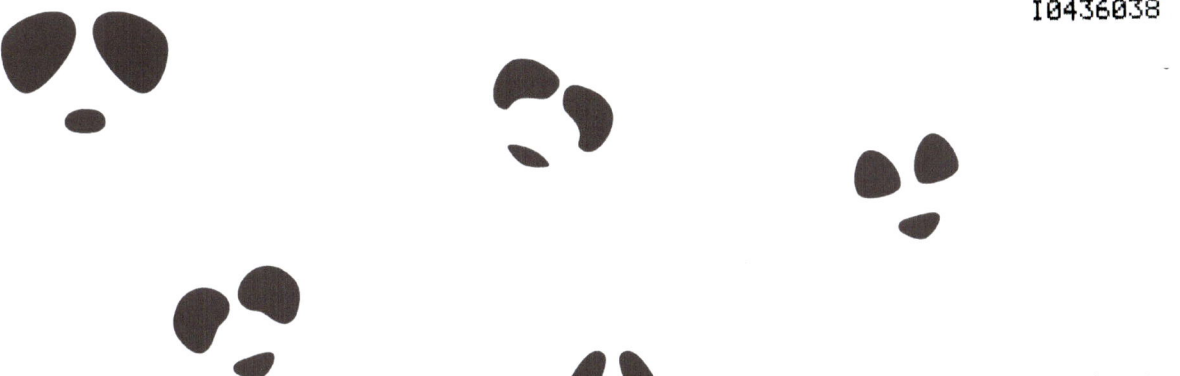

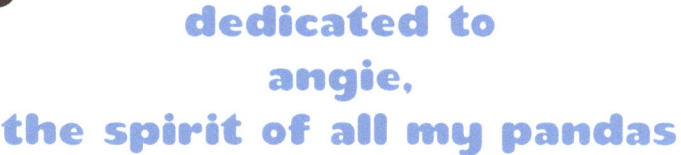
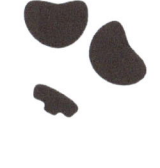

dedicated to
angie,
the spirit of all my pandas

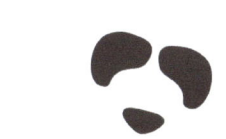

welcome to the world of

zen panda

i'm orin and i live
in an ancient panda village
deep in the forest. my tribe and i want
to share our secrets to being happy and
healthy everday.

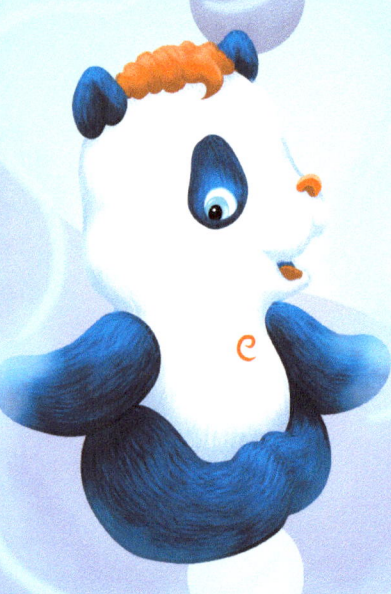

everyone in our village has different skills and
interests and these yoga poses help us be ready
to do great things each day. you can work
through all the poses in the book or only do the
short routine if you have less time (poses
marked with the lotus symbol).

just a few things to remember:

* bear feet on a mat is typically how we practice, but not required. just make sure your feet won't slip around

* do the warm-ups before each session

* focus on breathing in through your nose and out through your mouth slowly and evenly during poses

* poses may show a stretch with one leg or side of the body – remember to do those poses with both sides

* stretch only as far as it feels good – if it hurts you have pushed too far

* we are pandas and our bodies might look a little different than yours in some of the poses

* there is no failing – success is practicing poses everyday you can

* every body is different so focus on what feels right for you, not others around you

🔶 shoulder rolls

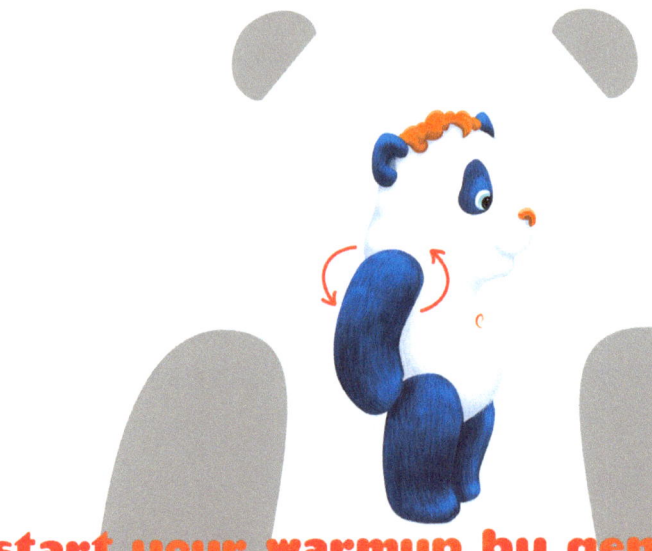

start your warmup by gently rolling both your shoulders up, around and down in a circle. do 10 circles, then reverse directions for 10 more.

🔶 windmills

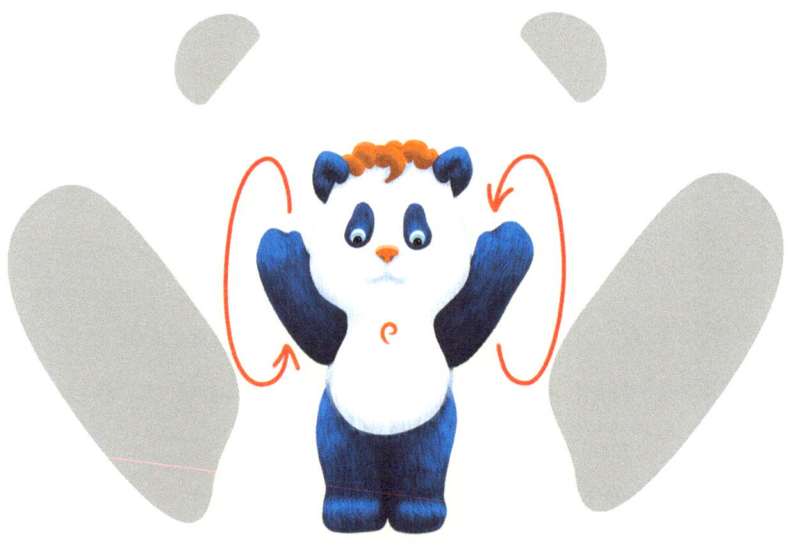

rotate your arms in circles as big as you can 10-15 times.

◉ hip rotation

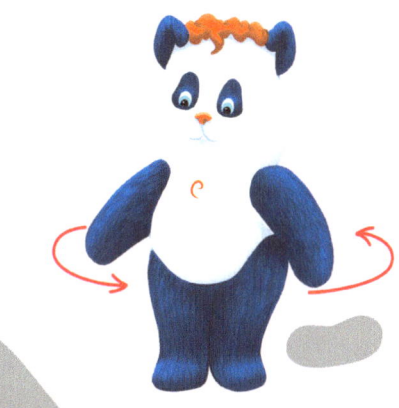

gently rotate your hips in a circle.
move slowly and remember to breathe.
do 10 circles and then reverse
directions for 10 more.

◉ torso twists

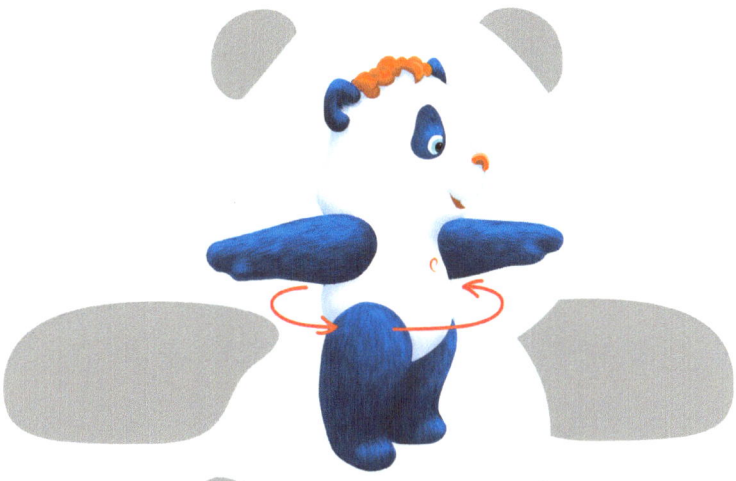

let your arms swing out as you gently
twist your torso from side to side. do 10
twists to each side.

◉ tadasana mountain pose

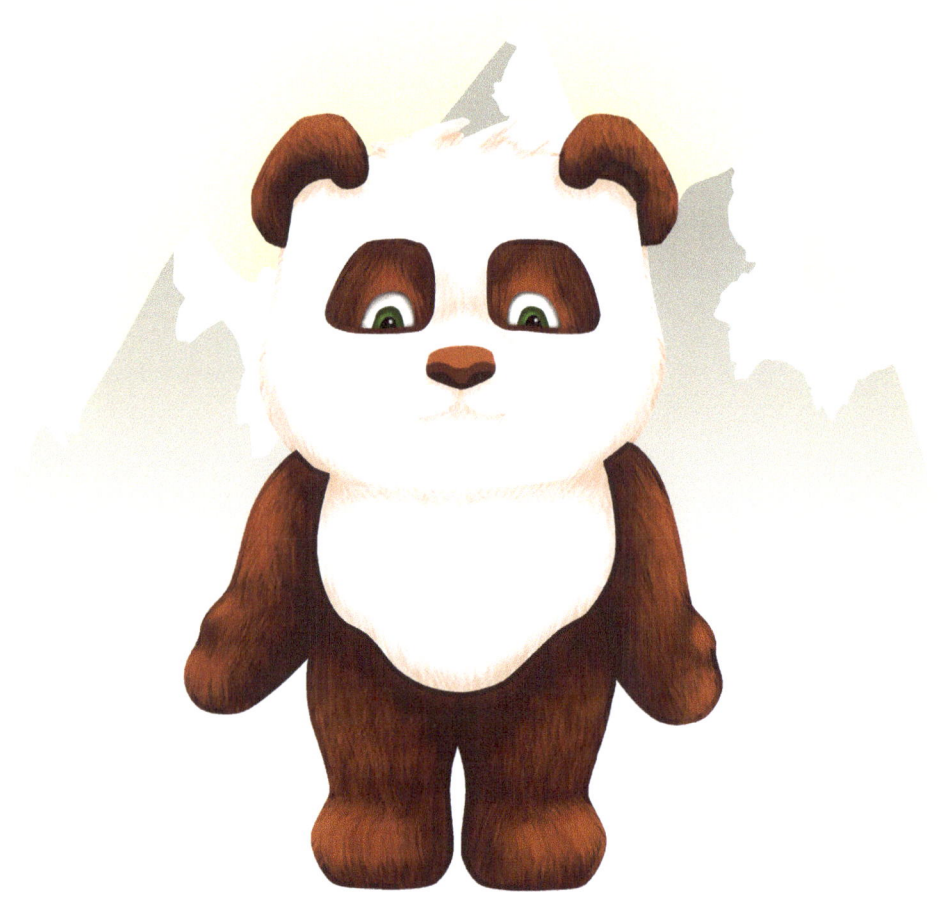

enu develops awareness of posture, promotes spinal alignment and focuses on his breathing in this basic standing pose.

virabhadrasana 2
warrior 2

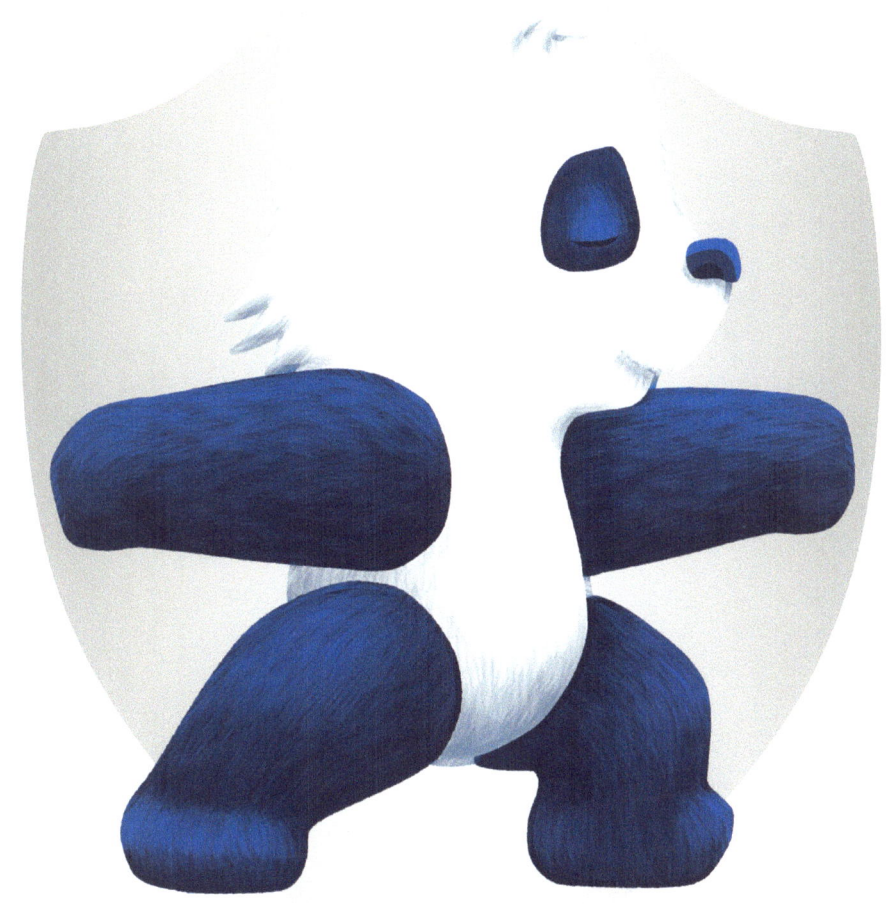

otoro expands his chest, strengthens his legs and back, and focuses his mind.

vrksasana
tree pose

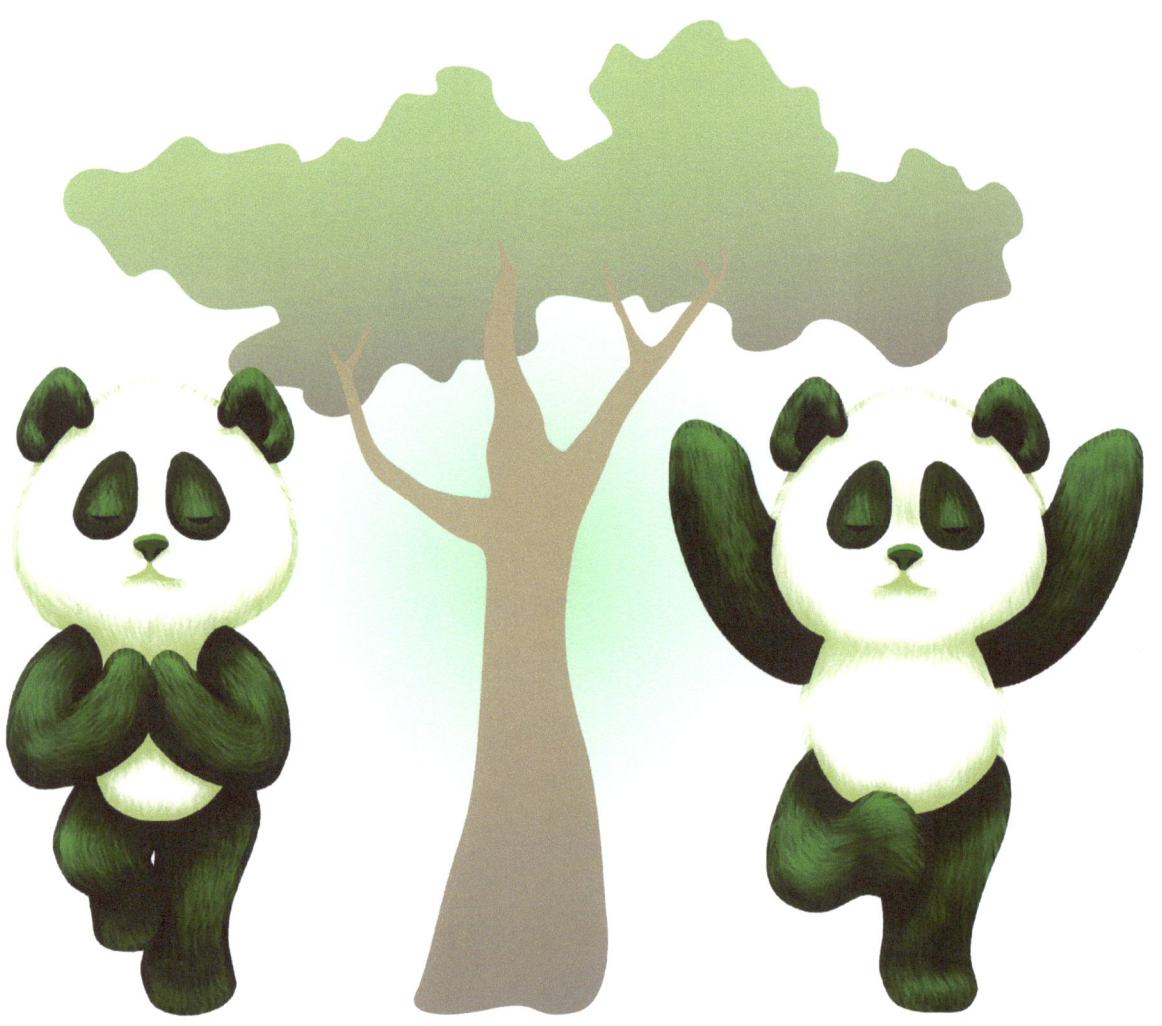

kani tones her legs in basic tree pose. with practice, she improves her balance and concentration and moves on to the advanced pose.

uttihita trikanasana
extended triangle

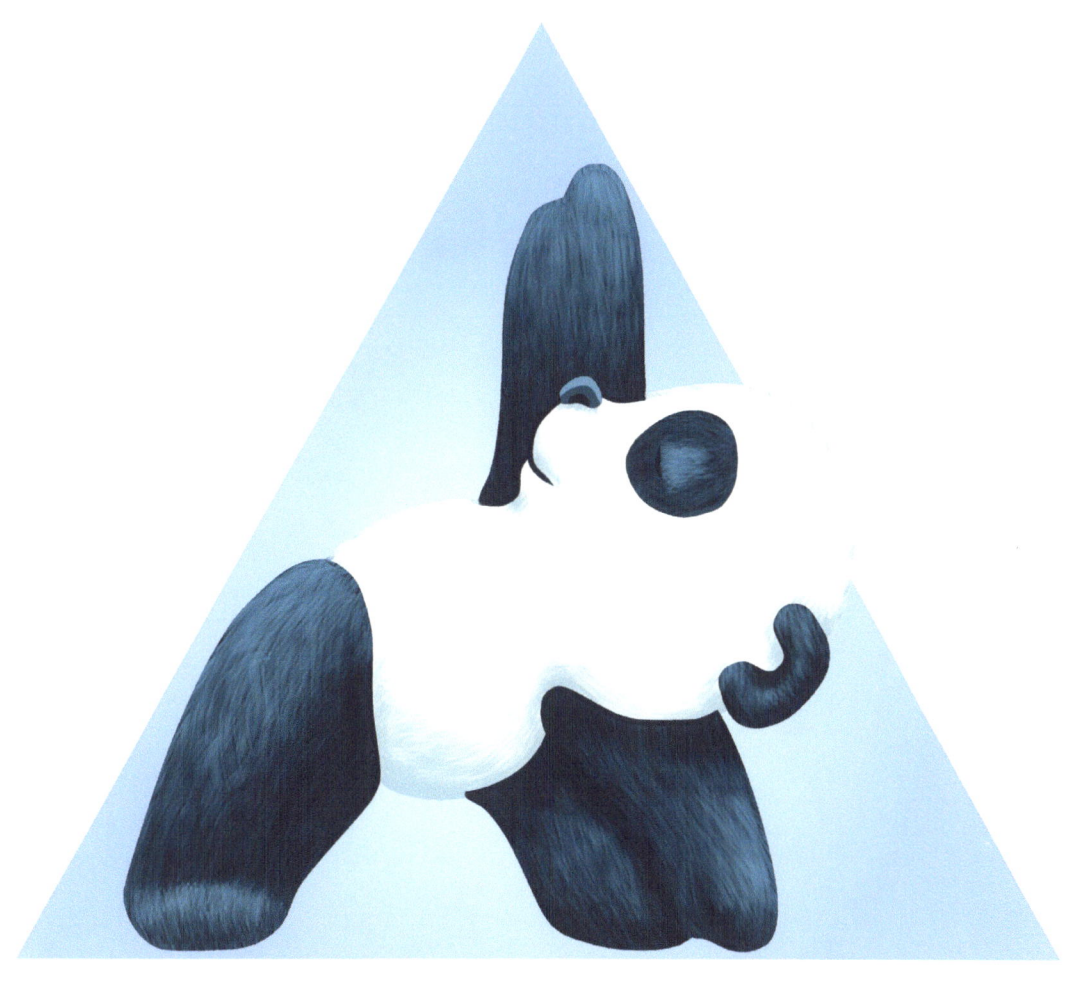

jala uses this pose to strengthen her ankles and legs for her training as a stone carver.

garudasana
eagle pose

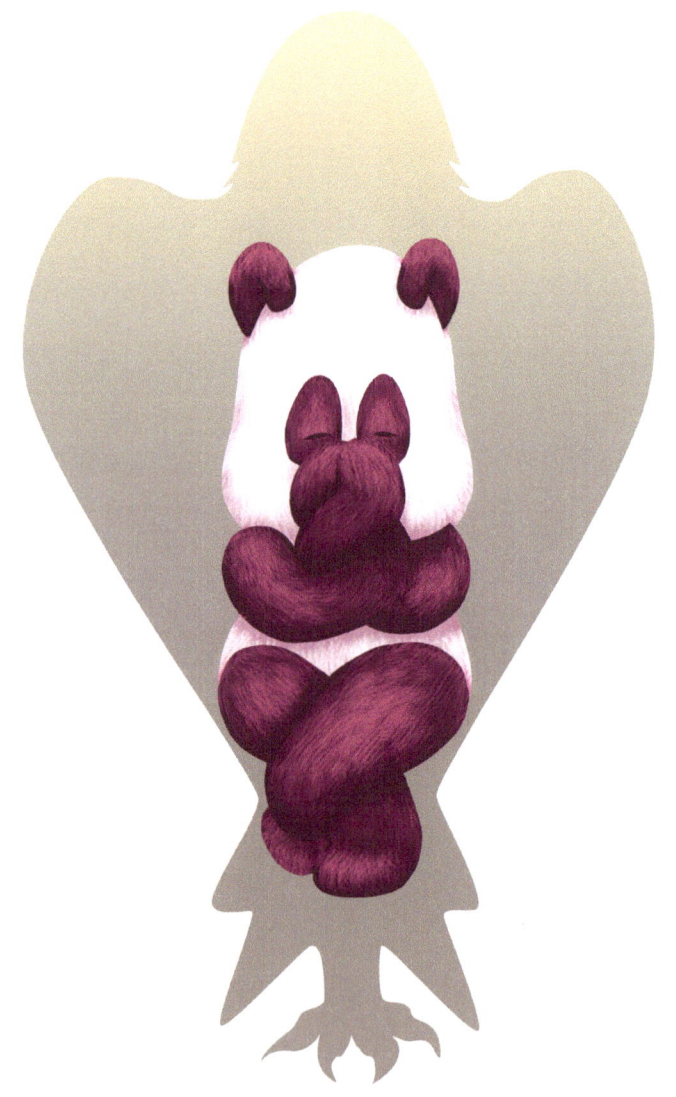

risha uses eagle pose to improve concentration and increase circulation, both which aid her skillful pottery and weaving.

⬡ baddha konasana
butterfly pose

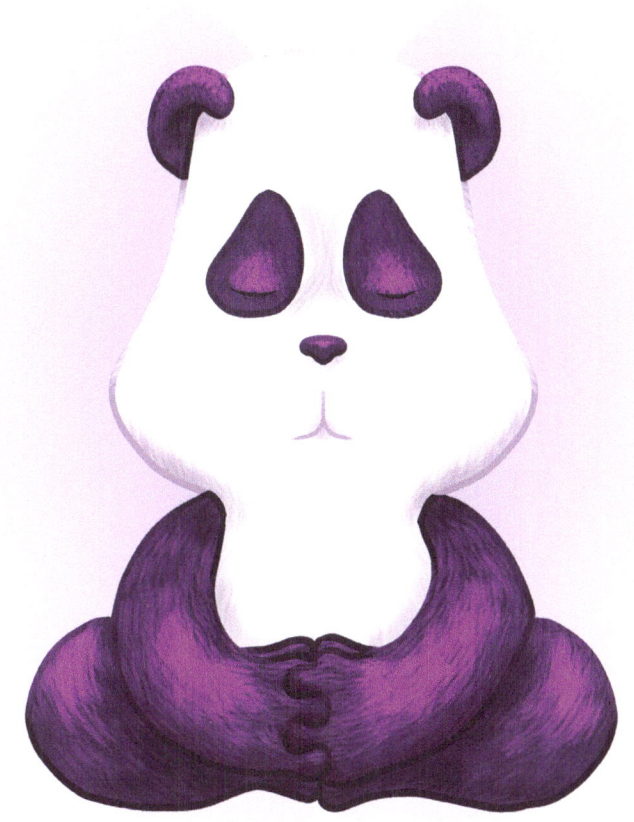

oimu uses this pose to increase her flexibility and tone her legs, increasing her stamina as a healer.

varjrasana
thunderbolt pose

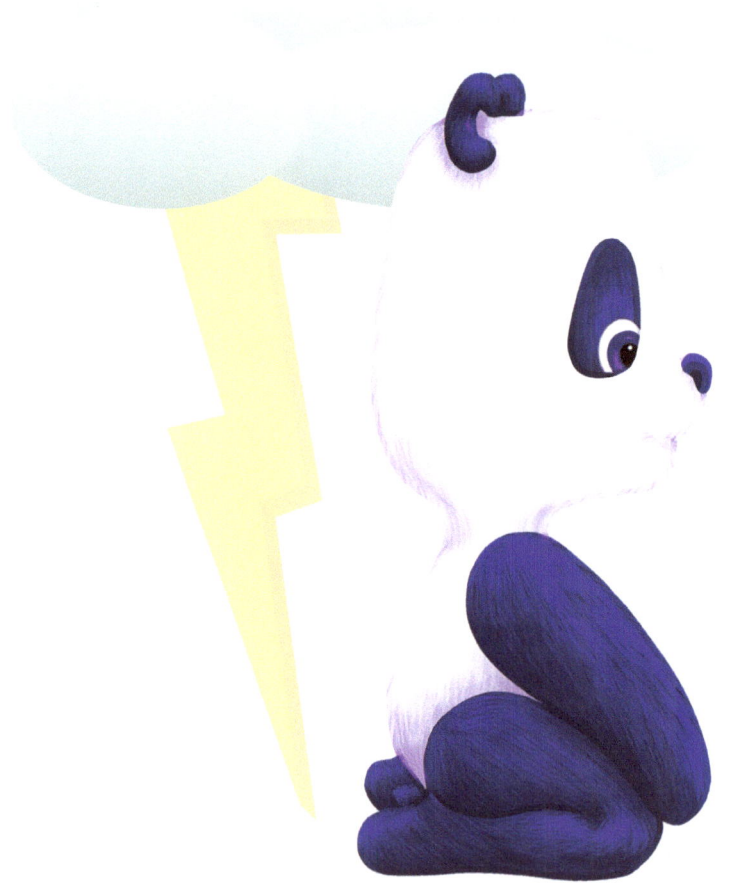

kino uses this pose to tone his legs and calm his mind to prepare for his training as a sky watcher.

ustrasana
camel pose

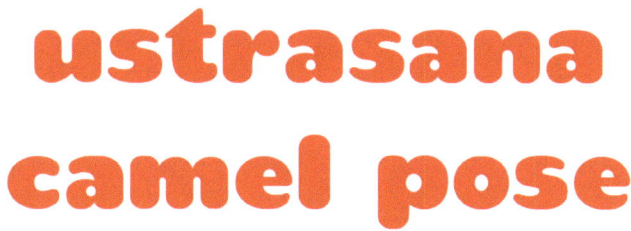

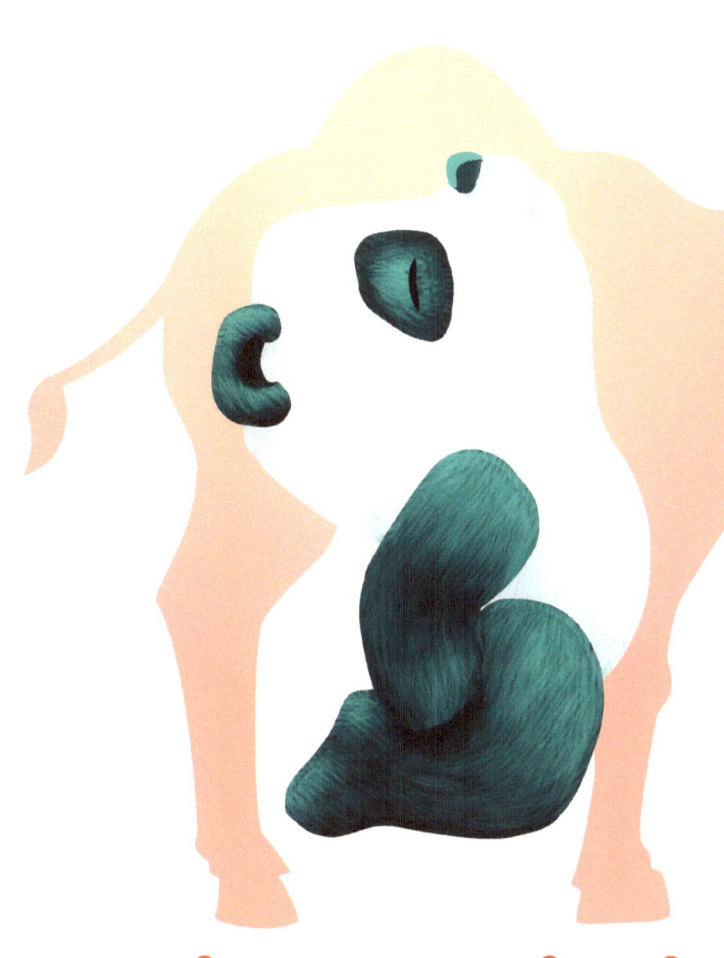

in camel pose, pulo cleanses his lungs and corrects the rounded shoulders he gets from training as a blacksmith.

anjaneyasana
crescent moon

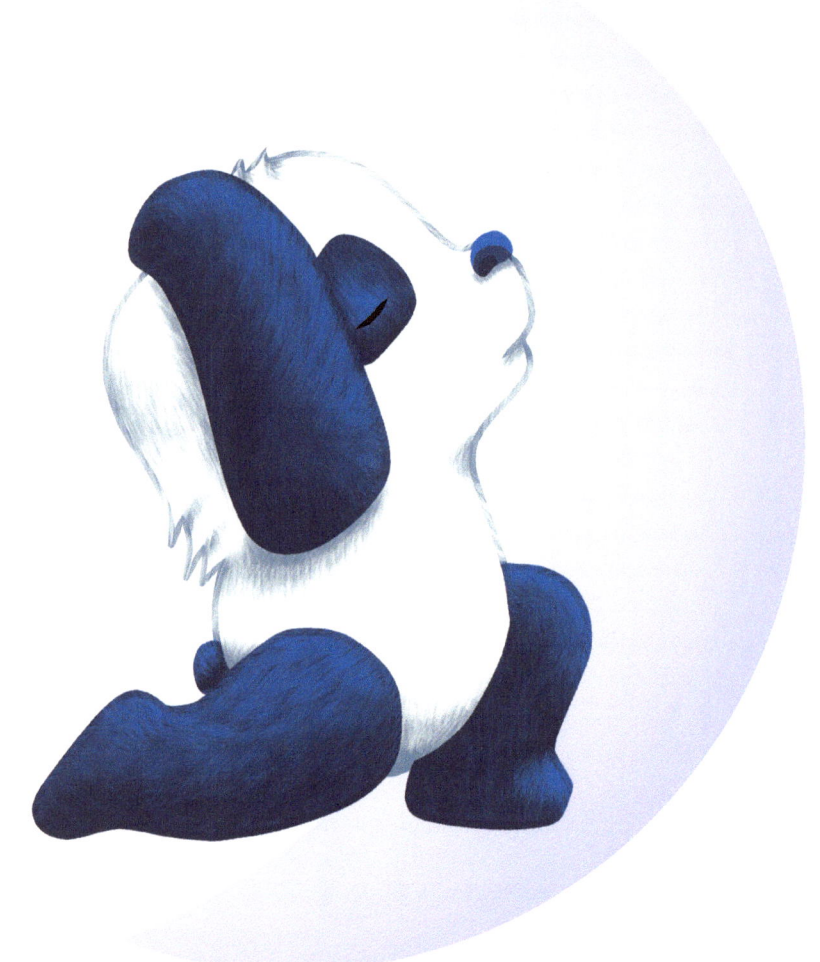

otoro strengthens his legs
and ankles with this pose
for all the patrols he walks
as a tribal guardian.

◉ nagasana
raised serpent

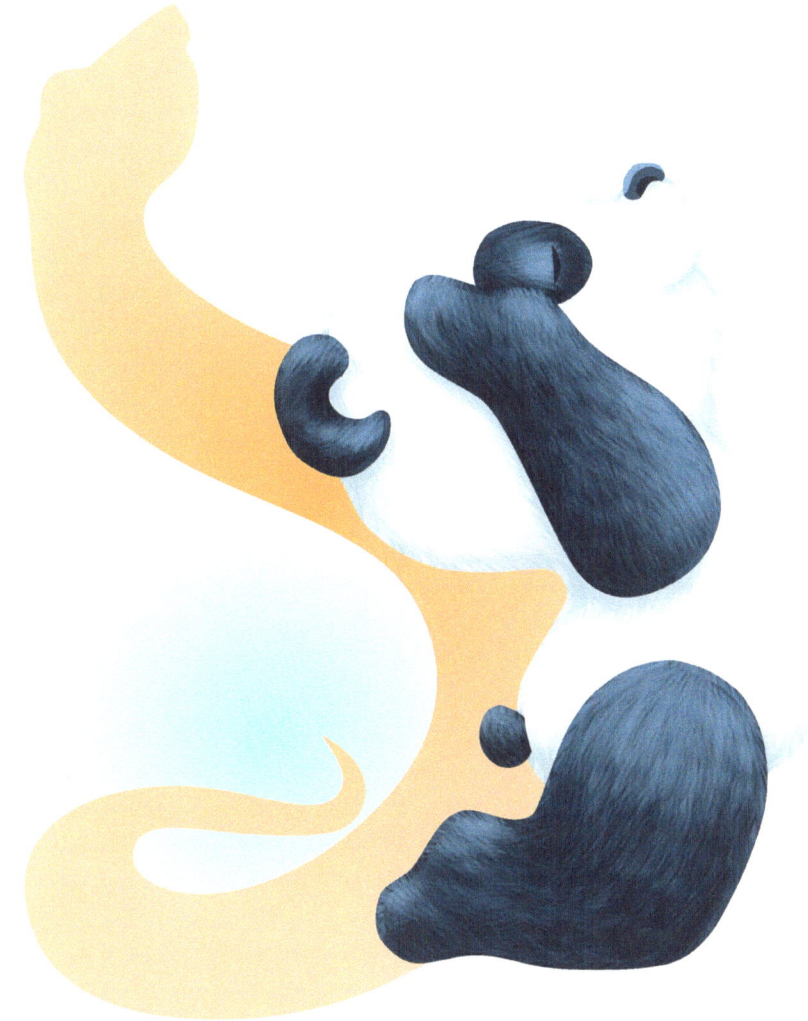

jala improves her posture and balance in raised serpent. it is also helpful to stregthen her knees, ankles, and spine.

⬣ hanumanasana
monkey pose

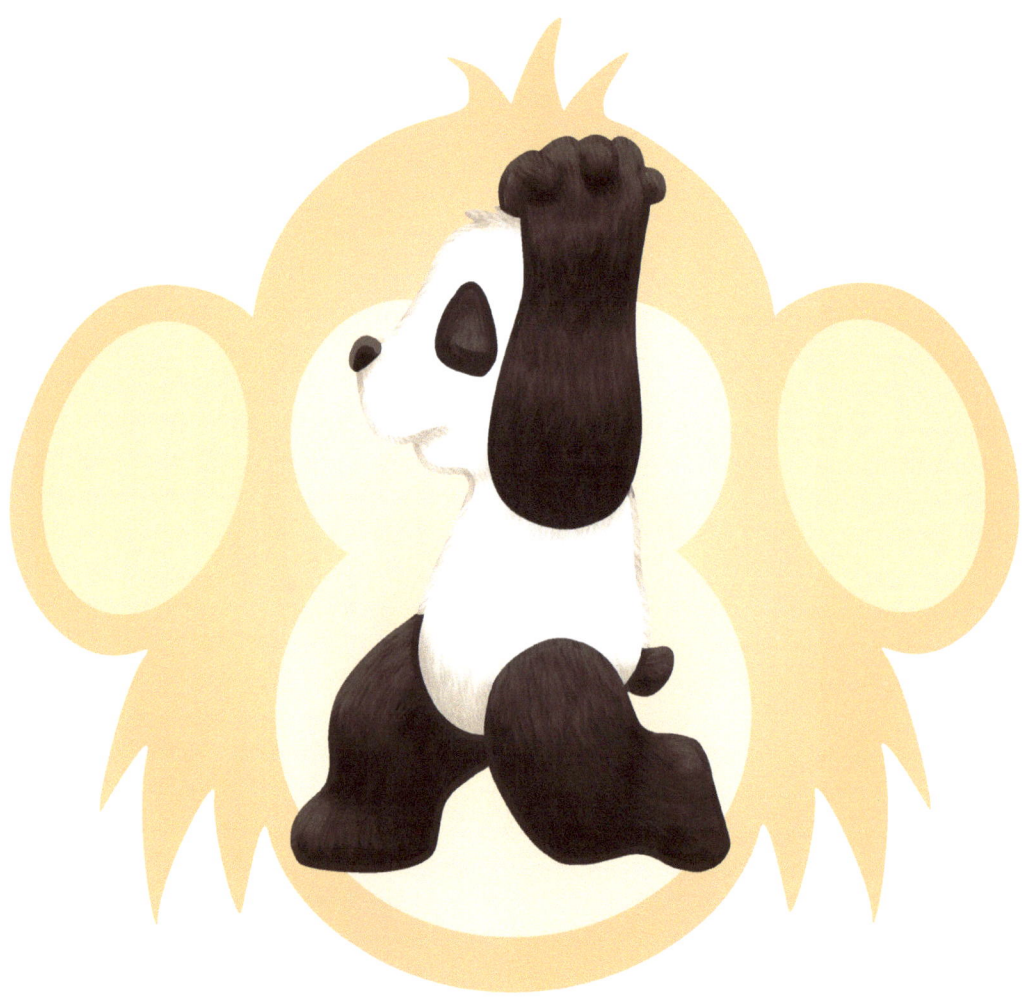

owaru tones his arms and legs and increases his flexibility at his hips to keep him patrolling as a warden of the wilds around his village.

adho mukha svanasana
downward dog pose

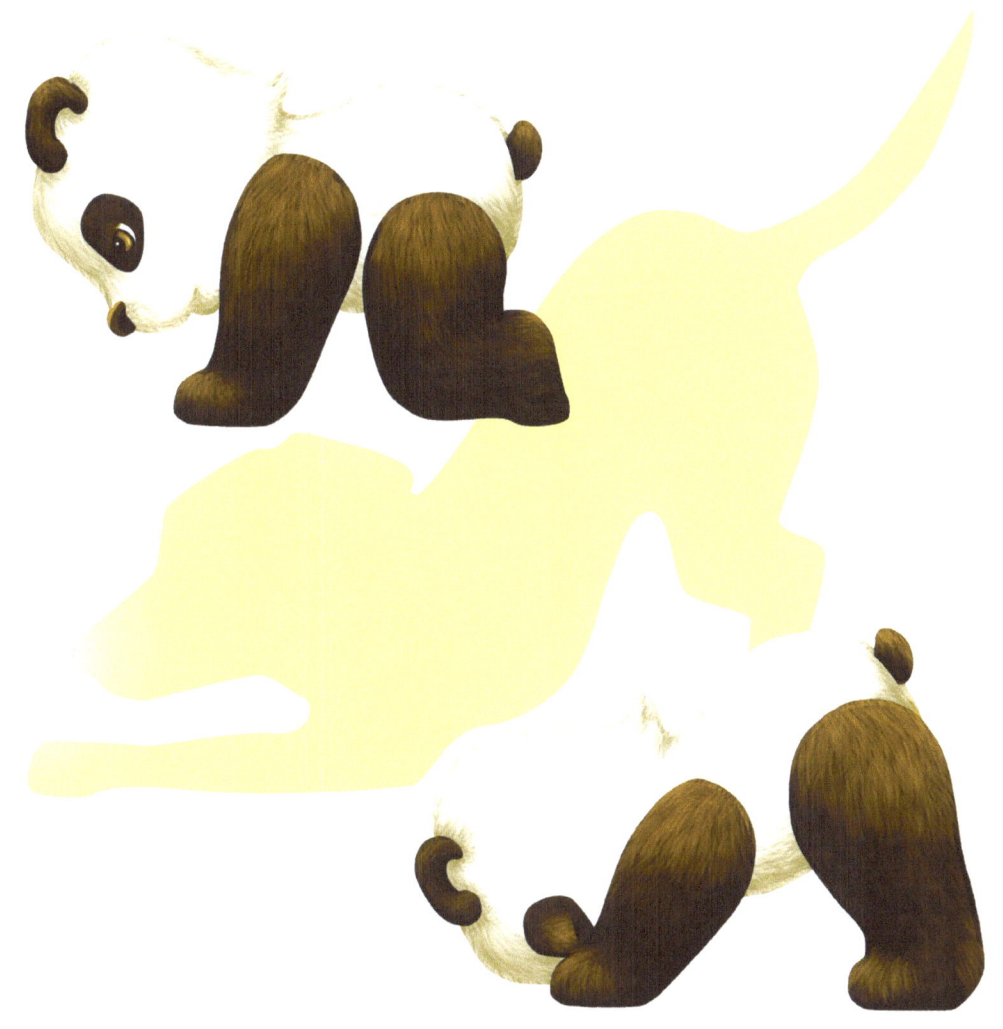

otine uses this pose to
stregthen and firm his
back, neck, core, and legs, as
well as restore his energy.

marjaryasana
cat pose

itori arches in cat pose to help keep his spine flexible and strengthen his back and pelvic area.

balasana
child pose

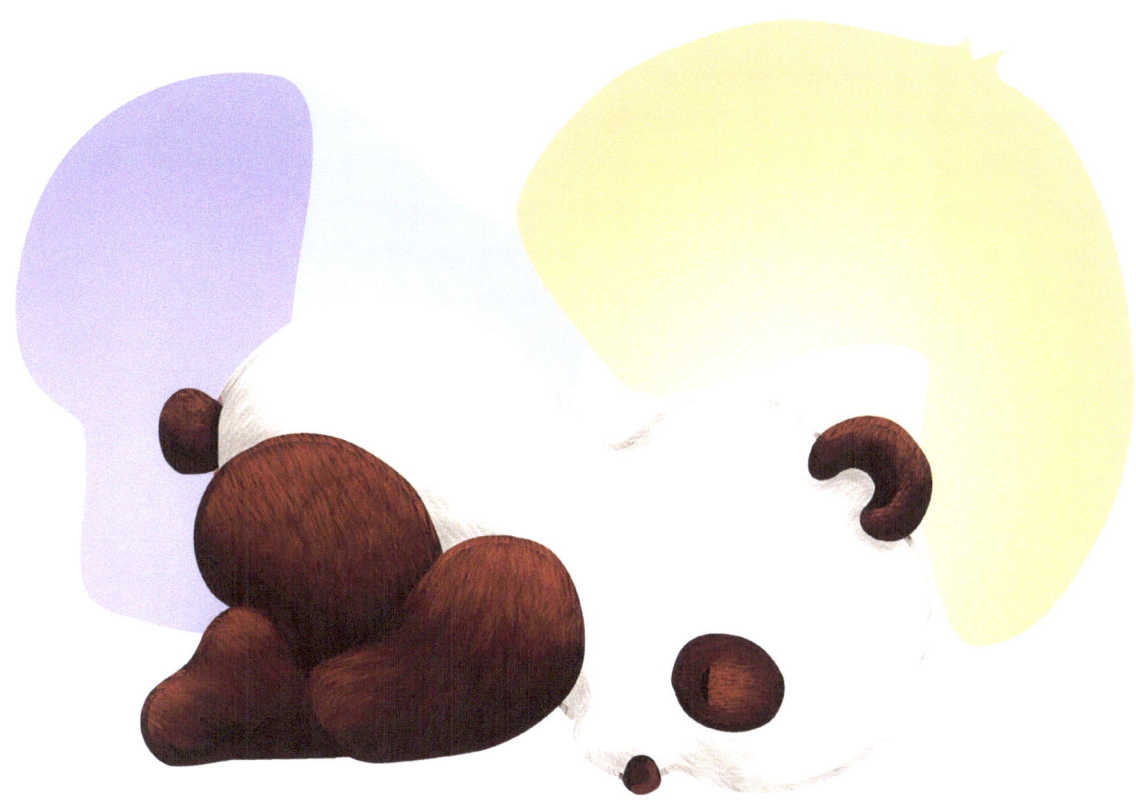

sero stretches his back, relaxes ligaments and reduces the fatigue he gets as a chef's apprentice.

sasamgasana
rabbit pose

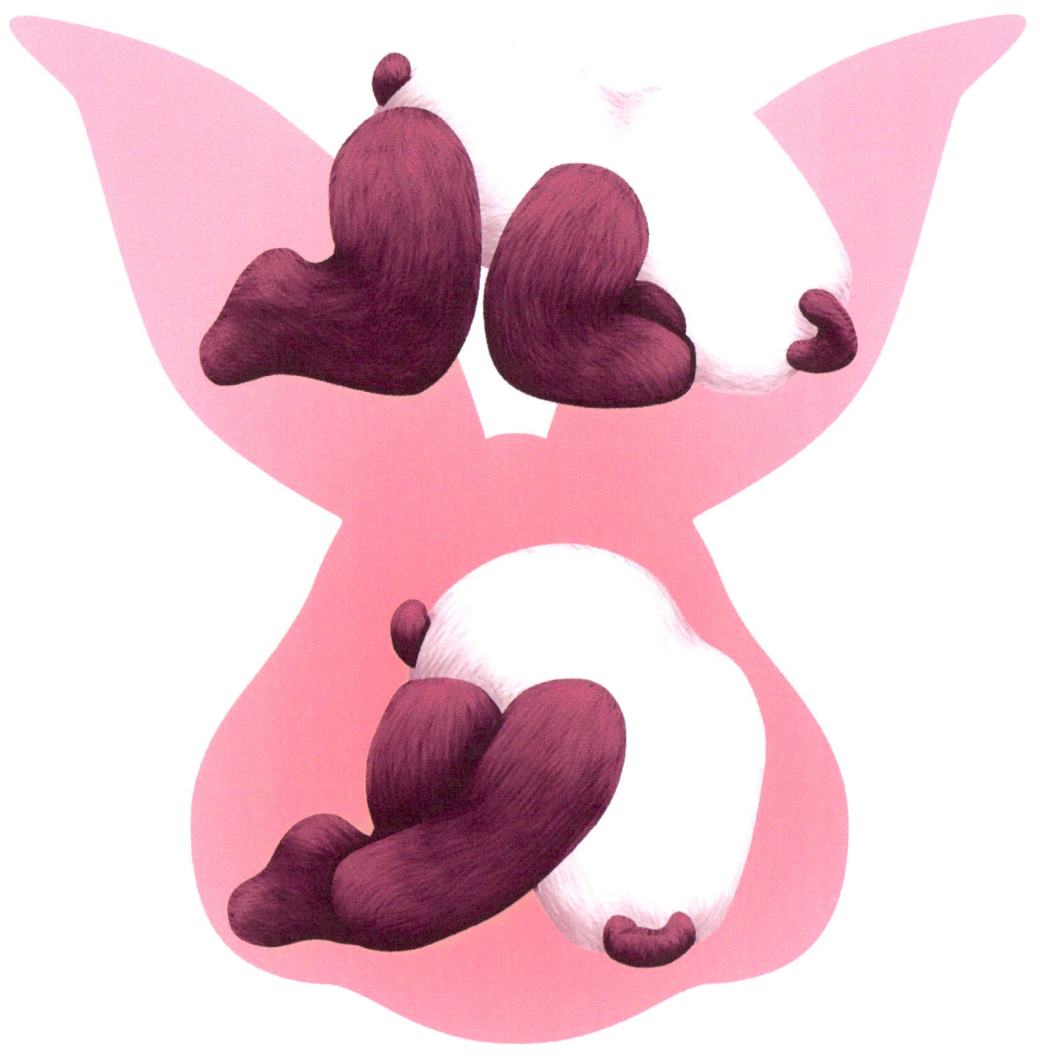

risha relaxes her shoulders
and refreshes her brain by
gently rolling into
rabbit pose.

bhujangasana
cobra pose

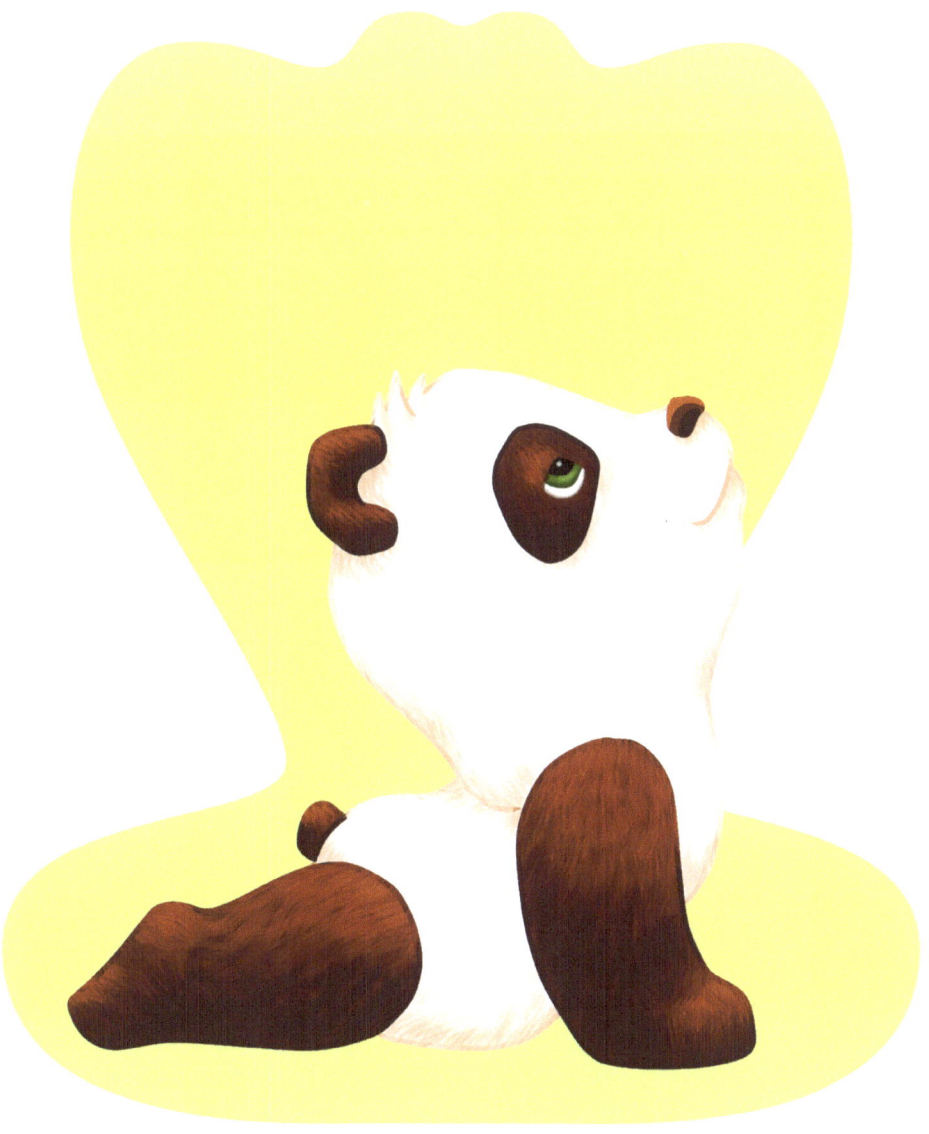

enu strengthens his back
with cobra pose for his work
as a carpenter.

salabhasana
flying locust pose

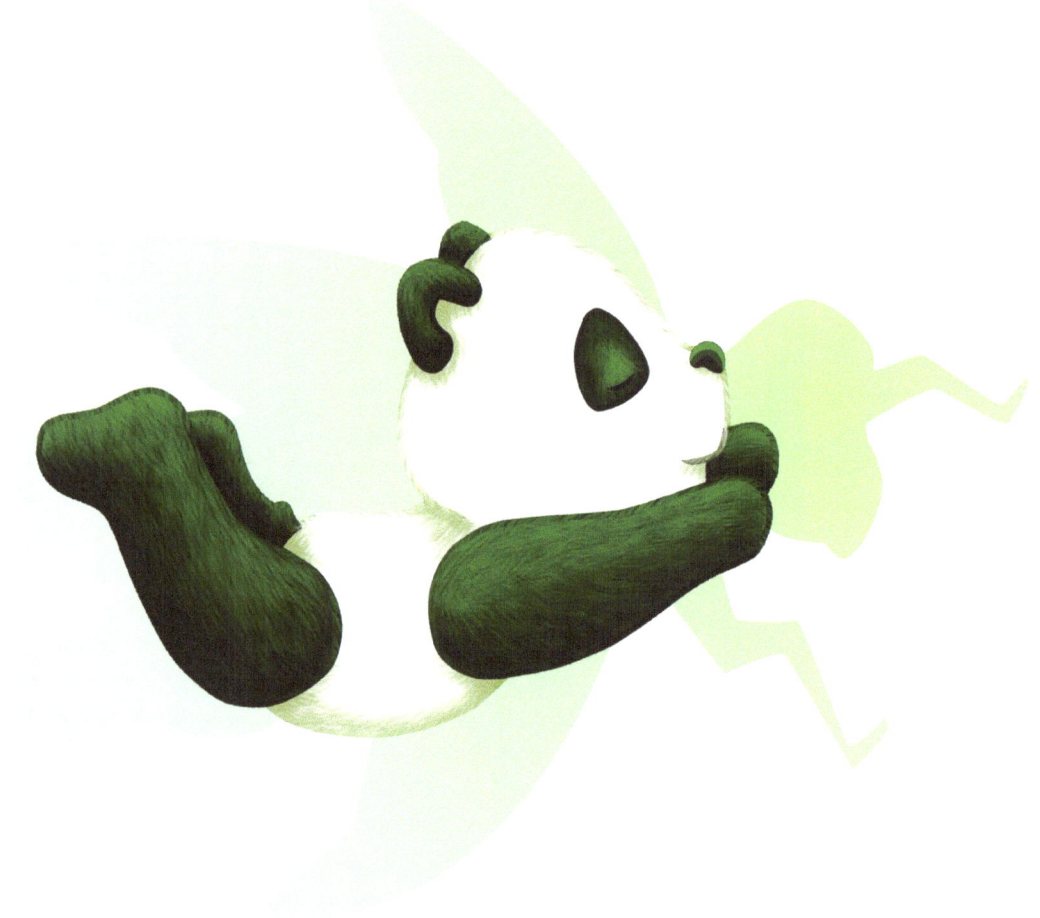

kani tones her shoulders, arms and legs. it also promotes the agility she needs to climb and scout the tree canopy around her village.

⬡ makarasana
crocodile pose

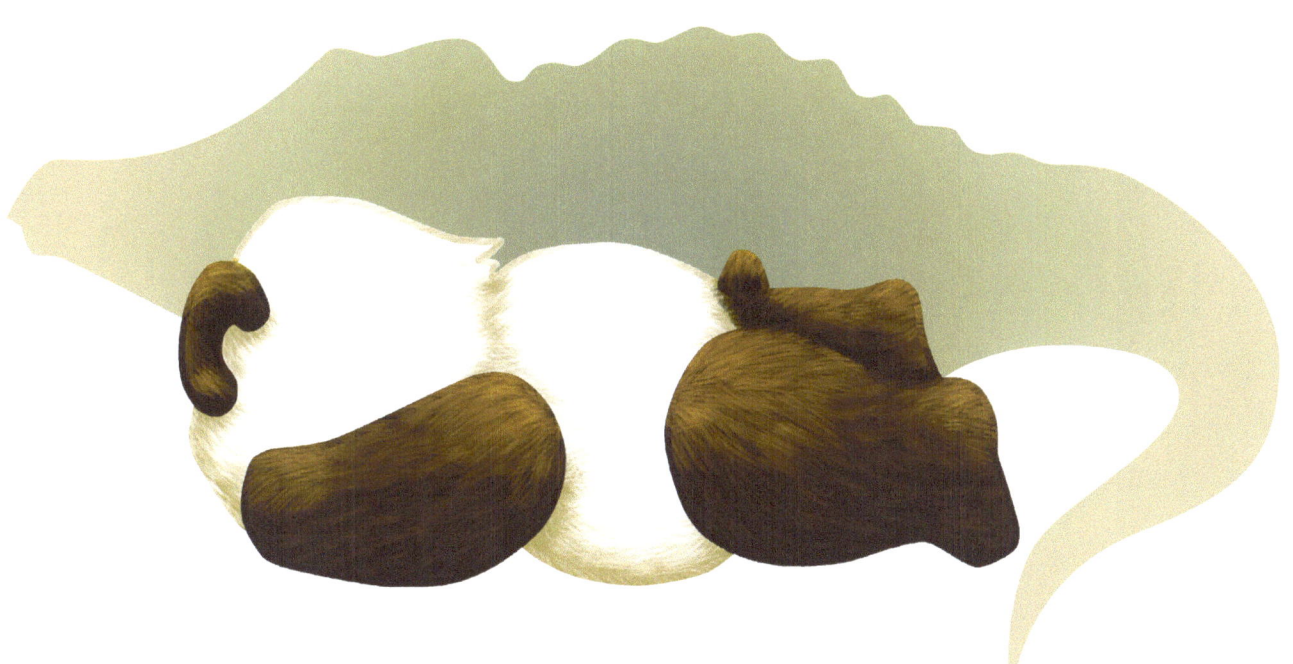

otine is a blacksmith and crocodile pose helps rest his body and quiet his mind after a hard day's at the bellows.

matsyasna
fish pose

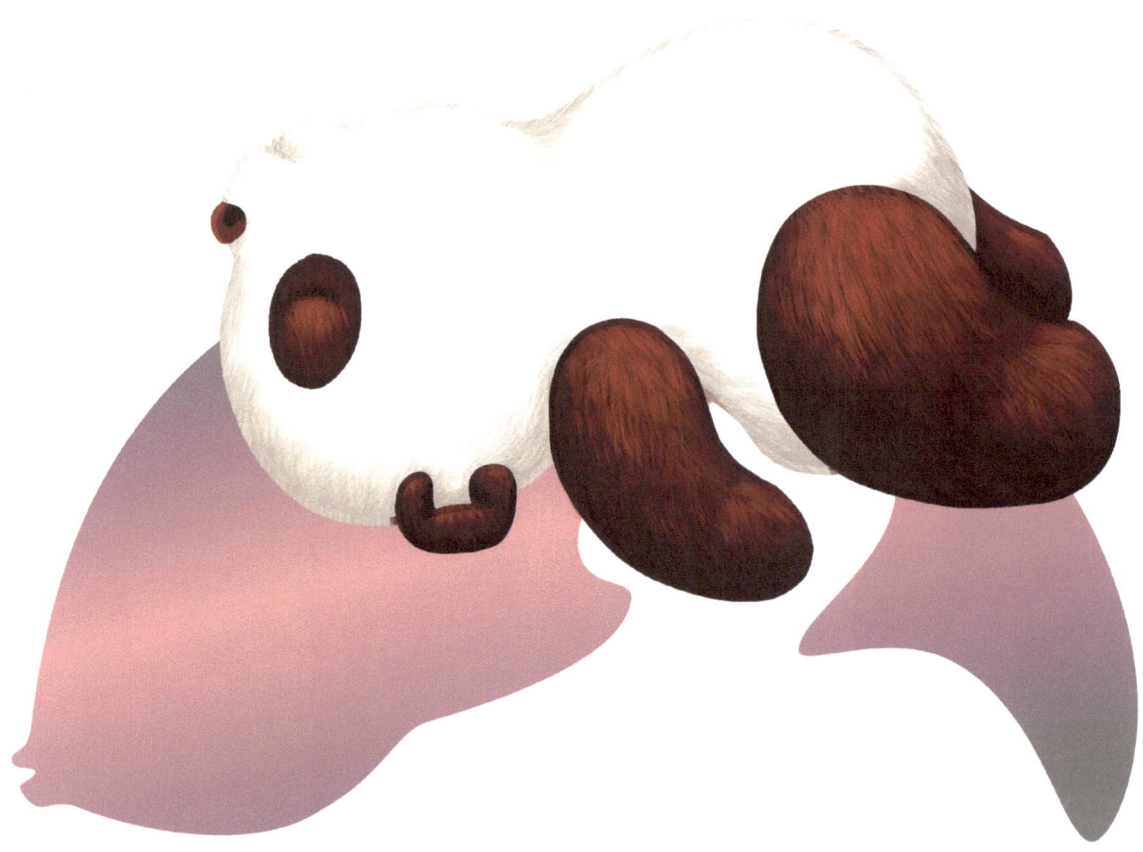

in fish pose, sero deepens his breathing and releases tension in his neck and shoulders.

navasana
boat pose

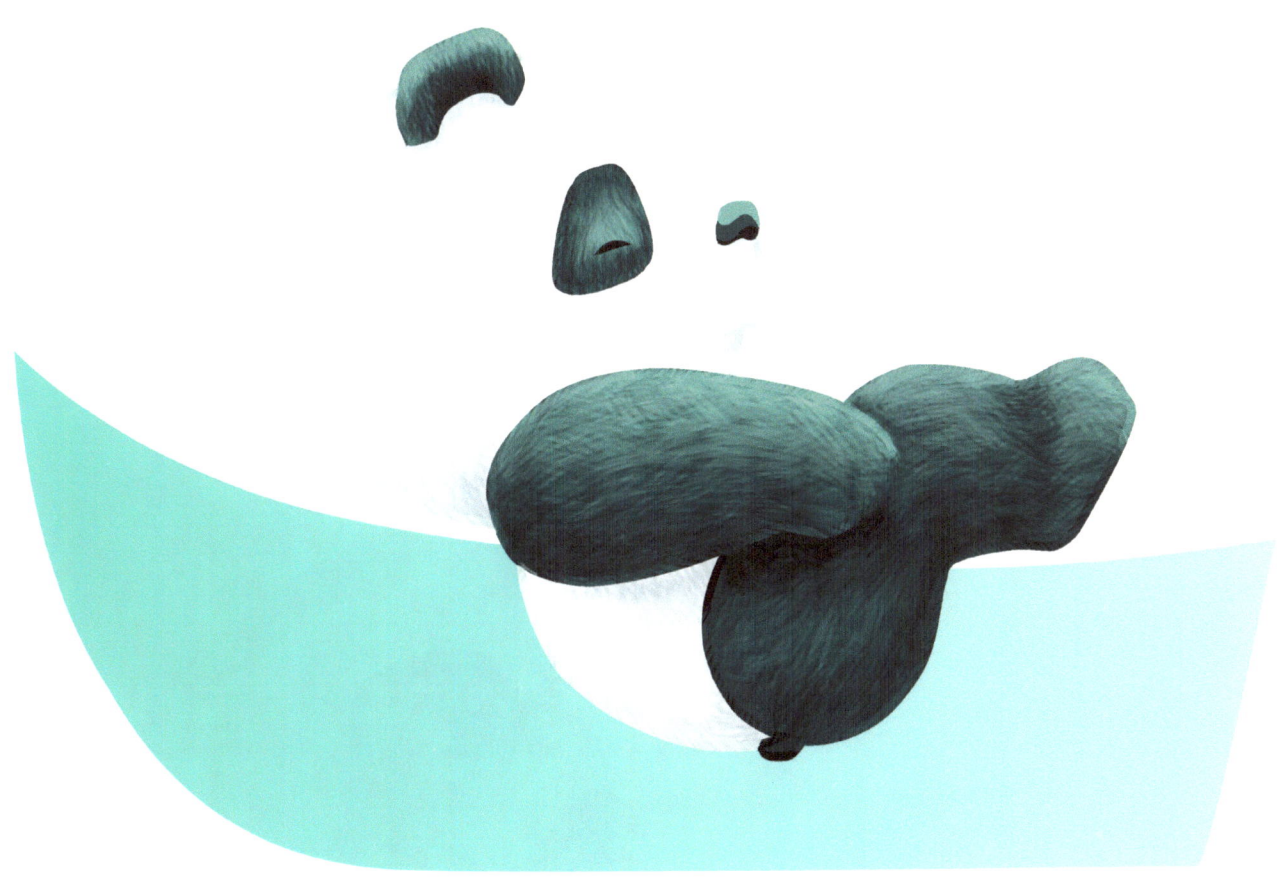

pulo strengthens the core muscles in his stomach by holding this pose.

setu bandhasana
bridge pose

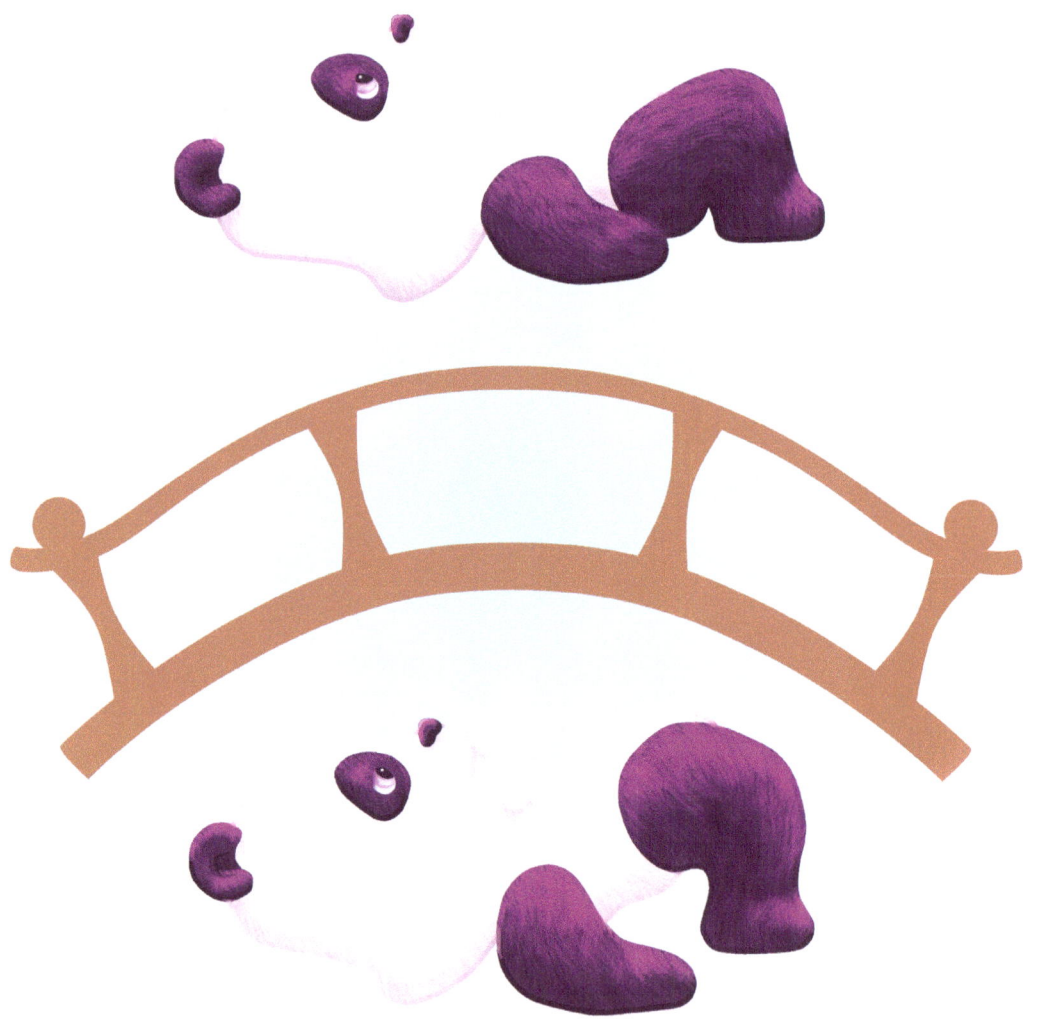

oimu flexes her spine and strengthens her wrists and ankles by holding the bottom pose.

ananda balasana
happy baby pose

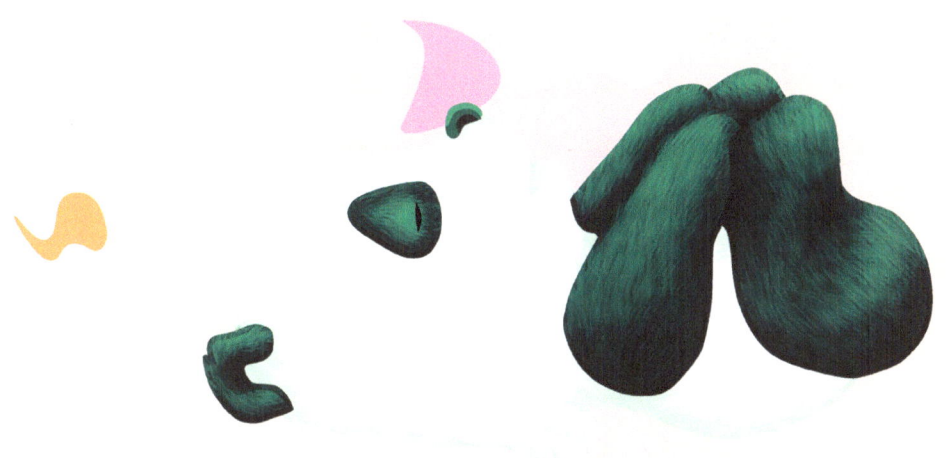

itori re-aligns his spine and stretches his hips when he relaxes into this pose. it also calms his mind after a day teaching the apprentices in his class.

pavanmuktasana
wind relieving

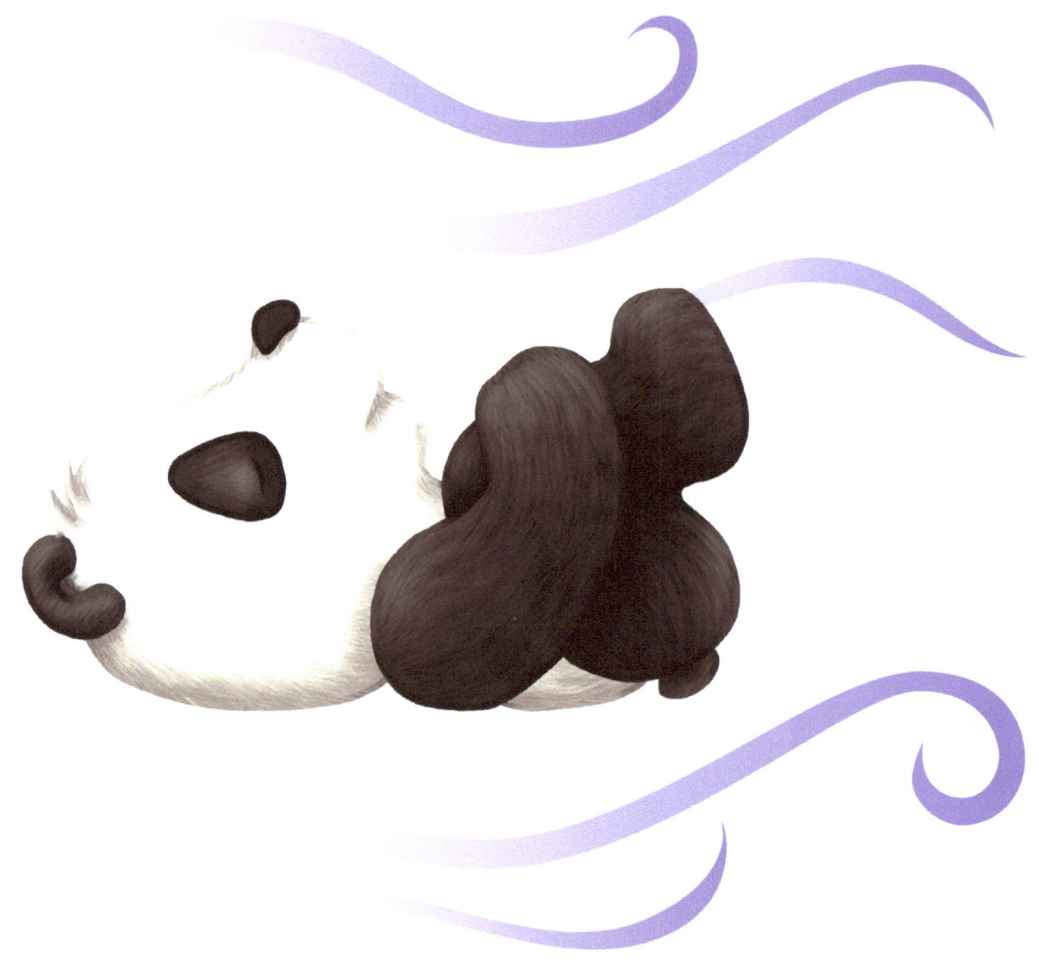

owaru limbers his spine,
hips and legs. he is also able
to cleanse his lungs and
release gas from his belly.

⬡ padmasana
lotus pose

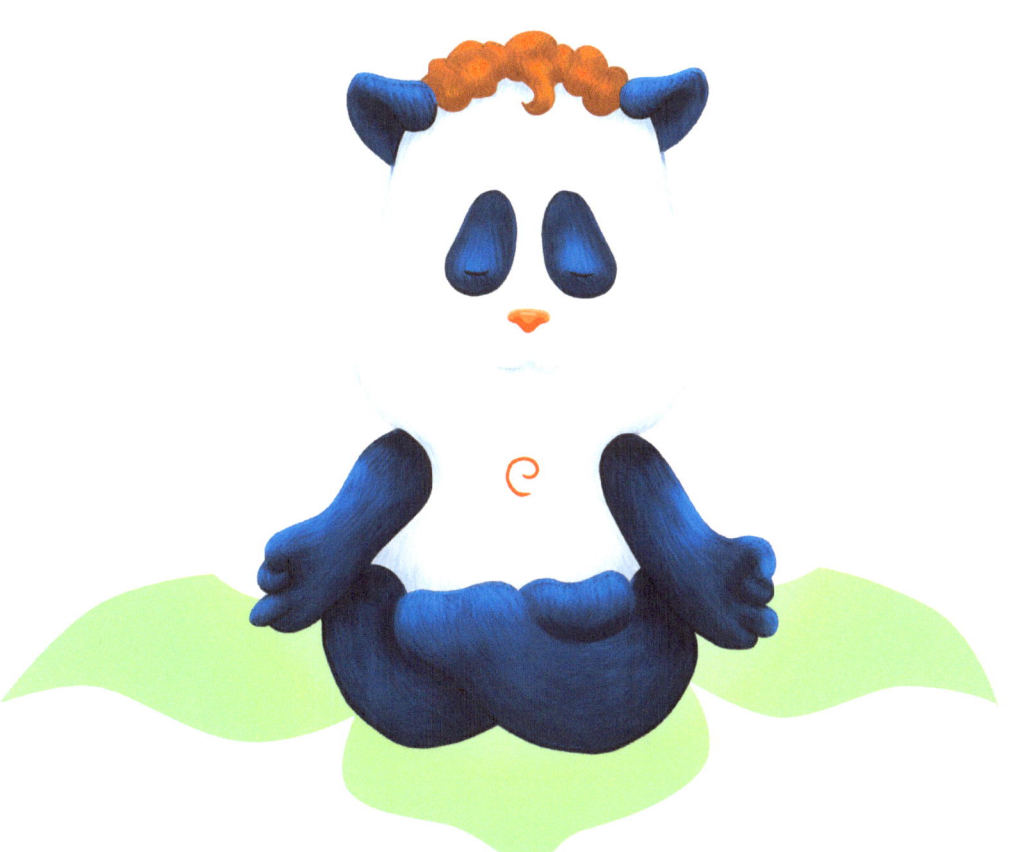

orin uses the full lotus to strengthen ankle, knee, and hip joints but can leave her feet on the floor if the stretch is too much.

◉ savasana
corpse - stillness

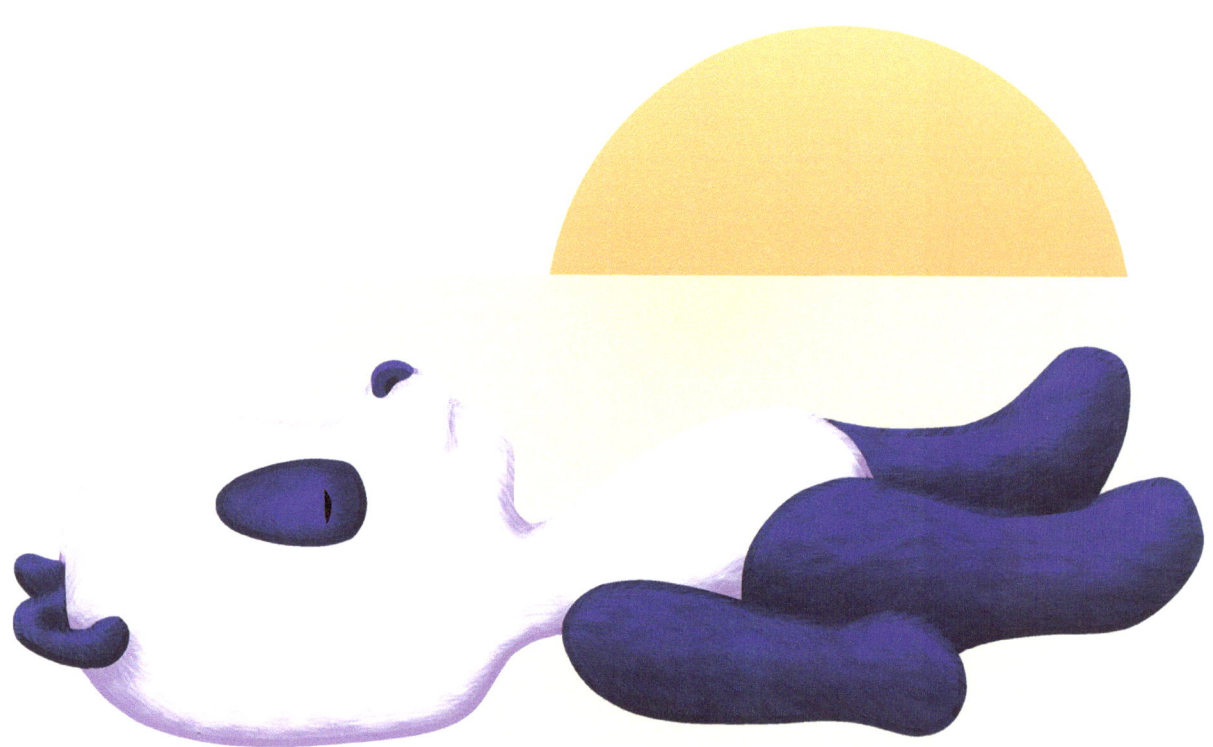

kino refreshes his mind and body by focusing on his breathing in this last pose of the session.

◉ namaste
i bow to you

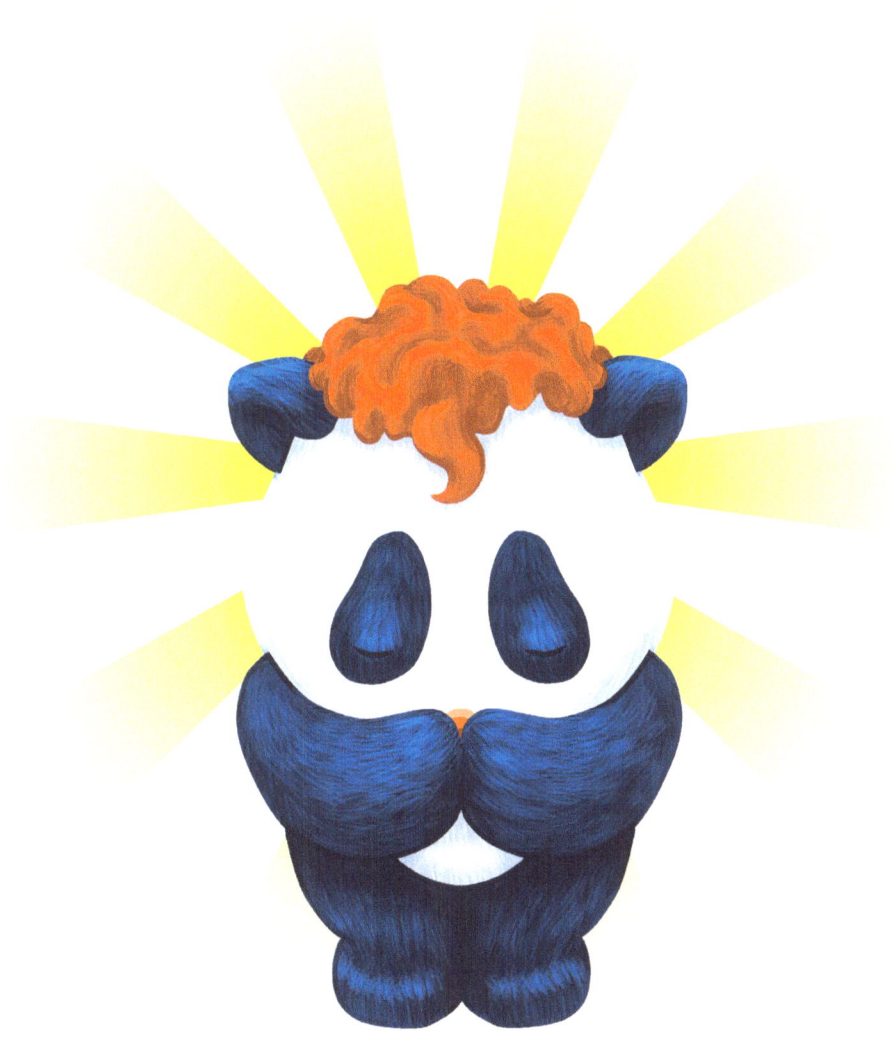

until we meet again.

www.ingramcontent.com/pod-product-compliance
Lightning Source LLC
Chambersburg PA
CBHW060811290526

45792CB00005BA/1606